AUTOPHAGY GUIDE

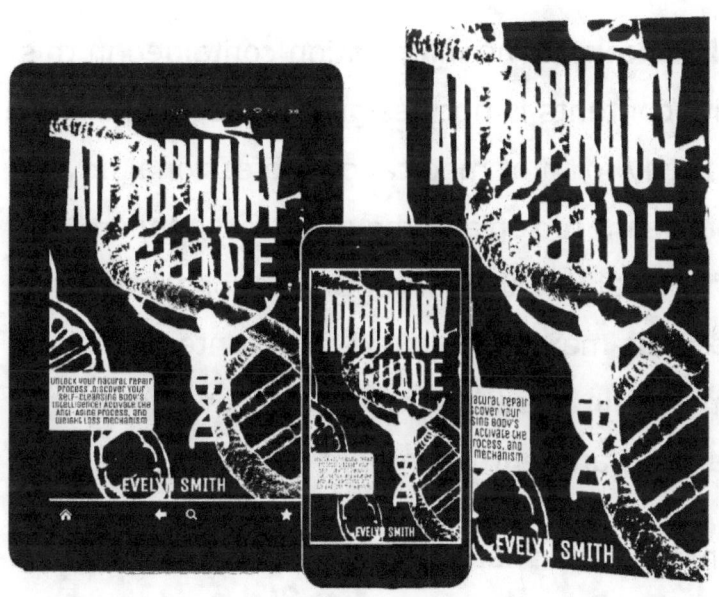

Unlock your natural repair process. Discover your self-cleansing body's intelligence. Activate the anti-aging process and weight loss mechanism.

Evelyn Smith

1

Legal & Disclaimer The information contained in this book and its contents is not designed to replace or take the place of any form of medical or professional advice; and is not meant to replace the need for independent medical, financial, legal or other professional advice or services, as may be required. The content and information in this book has been provided for educational and entertainment purposes only.

The content and information contained in this book has been compiled from sources deemed reliable, and it is accurate to the best of the Author's knowledge, information and belief. However, the Author cannot guarantee its accuracy and validity and cannot be held liable for any errors and/or omissions. Further, changes are periodically made to this book as and when needed. Where appropriate and/or necessary, you must consult a professional (including but not limited to your doctor, attorney, financial advisor or such other professional advisor) before using any of the suggested remedies, techniques, or information in this book.

Upon using the contents and information contained in this book, you agree to hold harmless the Author from and against any damages, costs, and expenses, including any legal fees potentially resulting from the application of any of the information provided by this book. This disclaimer applies to any loss, damages or injury caused by the use and application, whether directly or indirectly, of any advice or information presented, whether for breach of contract, tort, negligence, personal injury, criminal intent, or under any other cause of action.

You agree to accept all risks of using the information presented inside this book.

You agree that by continuing to read this book, where appropriate and/or necessary, you shall consult a professional (including but not limited to your doctor, attorney, or financial advisor or such other advisor as needed) before using any of the suggested remedies, techniques, or information in this book.

Table of Contents

Introduction

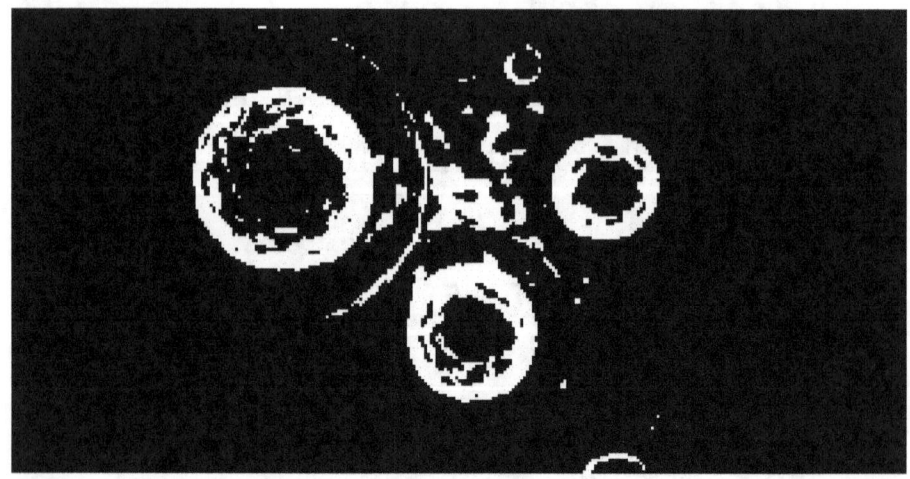

Autophagy is a natural process that occurs in our bodies continuously from birth. Our bodies use this process to recycle cells and their components. But even though autophagy is a cleanup process that happens all the time, now we have the knowledge to harness its power and tap its benefits when we want to. In the following article, we explain what autophagy is, and how to induce it when you want to experience its benefits.

What is autophagy?

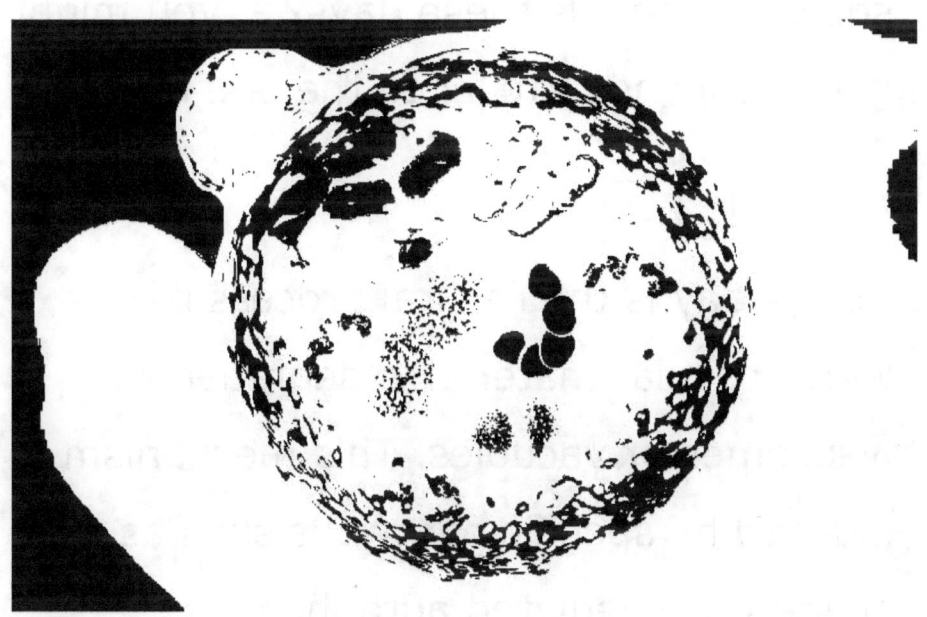

You might have heard of autophagy before. You might even know people who say that this process helped them lose weight. But how can autophagy help someone lose weight since it's basically a natural cleaning process? Let's find out.

The Autophagy Definition

If you pick up a biology manual or look up autophagy in search engines – do people still use manuals these days? -, you might get a response similar to the one below:

Autophagy is the natural process by which cellular material is degraded by lysosomes or vacuoles. This mechanism is induced by specific pathways such as chaperone-mediated autophagy, macroautophagy, and microautophagy. Now, this definition is very technical, but it's also very difficult to understand. Sure, we might understand some of the words, but what do they actually mean? Let's break it down.

Autophagy is a process in which cells eat themselves (in Greek, the term literally means self-eating). All cells degrade at certain rates. For example, a red blood cell lives on average 115 days. The cells on the top layer of our skin usually live 14 – 30 days, whereas neurons can live for years.

But the human body is extremely efficient, and it doesn't want to lose all the components of the dead cells, or the damaged components of living cells only to create them again from scratch for new cells that serve the same purpose.

This is where the lysosomes come in. These organelles break down the cells and they recycle all the useful components like protein while eliminating intracellular pathogens such as bacteria or viruses. They dispose of the cells' dysfunctional parts. We'll talk more about why this important below.

Selective Types of Autophagy:

The focus of this special issue of the International Journal of Cell Biology is to underscore the recent developments in the field of macroautophagy and how this degradative pathway intersects with cellular metabolism, complex physiological functions, and human diseases. During the last decade, autophagy has become an expanding field in biomedical life sciences due to its involvement with numerous intracellular processes. Autophagy also plays a role in pathology, and it has the therapeutic potential to be the target for the treatment of specific human diseases. Early studies suggested that autophagy was a nonselective process in which cytoplasmic structures were randomly sequestered into autophagosomes before being delivered to the mammalian lysosome or the plant and yeast vacuole for degradation. Now there is growing evidence that unwanted cellular structures can be selectively recognized and exclusively eliminated within cells (F. Reggiori et al., "Selective types of autophagy"). This is achieved through the action of specific autophagy receptors, as reviewed by C. Behrends and S. Fulda in "Receptor proteins in selective autophagy") and studied by K. Marchbank et al. "MAP1B interaction with the FW domain of the autophagic receptor Nbr1 facilitates its association to the microtubule network". Thus excess or damaged organelles including mitochondria (A. May et al., "The many faces of mitochondrial autophagy: making sense of contrasting observations in recent research"; Y. Hirota et al., "The physiological role of mitophagy: new insights into phosphorylation events"), peroxisomes (A. Till et al., "Pexophagy: the selective degradation of peroxisomes"), lipid droplets (R. Singh and A. Cuervo, "Lipophagy: connecting autophagy and lipid metabolism"), endoplasmic reticulum and ribosomes (E. Cebollero et al., "Reticulophagy and ribophagy: regulated degradation of protein production factories") can be specifically sequestered by autophagosomes and targeted to the lysosome for degradation.

Importantly, there is growing evidence that selective autophagy subtypes also have a wide range of physiological functions. In yeast, the cytosol-to-vacuole (Cvt) pathway transports hydrolases into the vacuole, which is reviewed by M. Umekawa and D. Klionsky in "The cytoplasm-to-vacuole targeting pathway: a historical perspective". In eukaryotes, autophagy plays a central role in both innate and acquired immunity. Further sequestration and elimination of invading pathogens such as Salmonella and Staphylococcus aureus have been exploited to study autophagosome biogenesis (T. Noda et al., "Three-axis model for Atg recruitment in autophagy against Salmonella"; M. Mauthe et al., "WIPI-1 positive autophagosome-like vesicles entrap pathogenic Staphylococcus aureus for lysosomal degradation"). In pancreas cells, autophagy has recently been shown to specifically turn over secretory granules, as described by M. Vaccaro in "Zymophagy: selective autophagy of secretory granules". Dysregulation of autophagic function has been implicated in a growing list of disease processes and has underscored the selective or substrate-specific versions of the pathway. Examples in this special issue include the clearance of aggregates associated with neurological diseases, as reviewed by T. Lamark and T. Johansen in "Aggrephagy: selective disposal of protein aggregates by macroautophagy" and by I. Nezis in "Selective autophagy in Drosophila". In terms of cancer biology, autophagy has been viewed as having dual roles in both tumor suppression and progression. K. Hughson et al. in "Implications of therapy-induced selective autophagy on tumor metabolism and survival" review how activation of autophagy selective forms can be used as a potential therapeutic approach for the treatment of specific cancers. Adding to the complexity of autophagic function and regulation, the article by K. Juenemann and E. Reits "Alternative macroautophagic pathways" explores alternative macroautophagic pathways that are independent of key core autophagy components such as Beclin-1 or Atg5. We expect future research on the mechanism and regulation of selective autophagy, and the physiological importance of this pathway in human disease will be very exciting and expand on the findings highlighted in this issue of IJC

The History of Autophagy

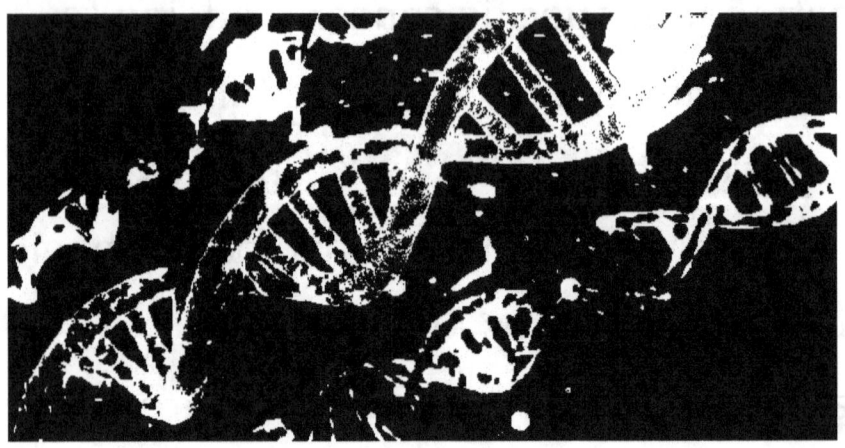

In 1963, Christian de Duve, a Belgian scientist was studying the effects of insulin on the liver when he stumbled upon a process nobody has documented before. He noticed that some cells cannibalized parts of their own structure in a presumed cleanup process. Thanks to de Duve's findings, the connection autophagy – lysosome was made.

Even though the Belgian scientist's discovery happened in the '60s and had lead to de Duve's Nobel Prize in 1974, it wasn't until the '80s that researchers really understood its importance.

The breakthrough came in 1983 when Japanese biologist Yoshinori Ohsumi discovered that specific genes regulate autophagy. He discovered that autophagy doesn't happen without the help of these genes, which means that cells can't repair themselves and the body doesn't recycle as many components when the cell dies. This discovery led to Ohsumi's Nobel Prize in 2016 and an important Breakthrough Prize in Life Sciences in 2017.

The Possible Benefits of Autophagy

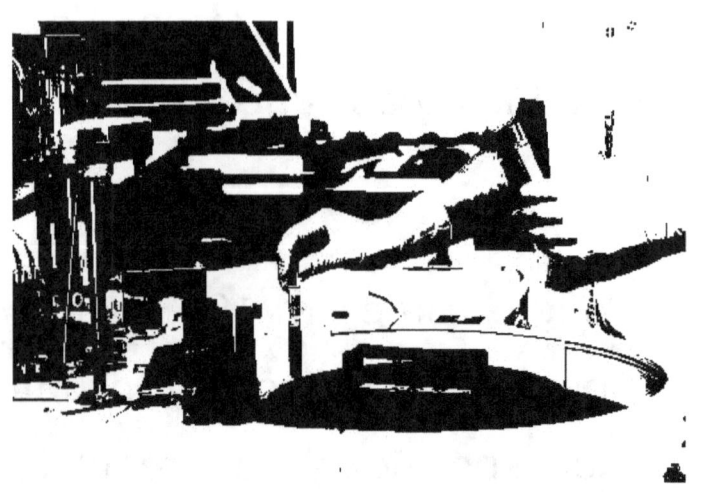

You might be wondering what makes autophagy so important. Well, according to the latest studies – and there have been thousands of articles published on autophagy until now – stimulating this process might produce a lot of benefits. Here is a list of the most important ones.

It May Extend Aging

Autophagy is important because it allows the body to reuse some of the cell's components, but it's also one of the ways the cell can actually repair itself. As cells age, they lose some of their functions. This is a natural process, one that's directly correlated to the cells' functional components. In truth, aging could be defined as the accumulation of different forms of molecular damage.

A cell accumulates its damaged components until a lysosome disposes of them. At the same time, the likelihood of developing chronic diseases such as diabetes or even cancer increases concomitantly with the accumulated damage.

By triggering the autophagy, the lysosome is removing the dysfunctional components, reducing their harmful potential. Since the cleanup process removes the damaged parts of the cell, it actually manages to prevent the development of diseases. And it gets better. Since aging could be defined as the sum of the cells' molecular damage, removing the damaged cells' components might actually delay the aging process itself.

Protects Against Psychiatric Disorders

Neurodegeneration is the leading cause of mental illness. And unfortunately, brain diseases are often difficult to treat. Neurons might be considered the most important cells in the body, but they still suffer damage every day. Sometimes, neural degradation is caused by the accumulation of proteins, while other times the neurons might be affected by a virus or bacteria. When a sufficient number of neurons are damaged, they start behaving erratically, leading to clinical manifestations of various psychiatric disorders.

However, recent studies suggest that autophagy might be an efficient way of preventing the onset of psychiatric diseases. Autophagy preserves the balance between the degradation of existing neurons, the recycling of their useful components, and the creation of new ones.

Those who suffer from schizophrenia show a deficiency in their autophagy pathways. Simply put, for those who suffer from schizophrenia, the autophagy process is not triggered at the right time. This creates an imbalance between the death of existing neurons and the creation of new ones, which leads to the disease's onset.

Prevents Neurodegenerative Disorders

You might have noticed that we talked about neural degradation caused by the accumulation of proteins. Well, this determines Alzheimer's, Parkinson's, and Huntington's diseases. The neurons of those who suffer from these diseases are assaulted by abnormal proteins called prions.

The accumulation of protein in the brain leads to profound changes in thinking and behavior and ultimately leads to the development of neurodegenerative diseases.

Autophagy increases the clearance of abnormal protein, as well as that of infectious and toxic agents. By triggering the autophagy process, researchers believe we might actually prevent the accumulation of both infectious and inflammatory agents that determine neurodegenerative diseases.

It Helps Fight Infectious Diseases

Autophagy can prevent the development of infectious diseases, and it can help fight the disease if you already contacted it. And the great thing is, this natural cleanup process is actually better at fighting infection than you would think.

You certainly heard of tuberculosis. Tuberculosis (or TB) is a disease that caused 1.3 million deaths worldwide in 2016 alone. You definitely know all about HIV, as well. These diseases are responsible for millions of deaths worldwide, and both of them can be prevented by autophagy.

When the lysosome triggers the autophagy mechanism, it targets the foreign and damaged components it finds in the cell for removal. The lysosome is so apt at removing the harmful components, it can degrade both the HIV virus and the TB bacteria so that they can't multiply and spread inside the body.

Regulates Inflammation

Autophagy helps regulate the body's inflammatory response. In fact, this is one of the mechanisms responsible for presenting the harmful particle to the immune cells which leads to the onset of the immune response.

And autophagy can also reduce the inflammatory response. All the foreign particles that enter the body are capable of launching an immune response. Even a damaged cell component can trigger an immune response if it's not cleared in a timely manner. By constantly removing these particles, the cleaning process helps regulate the inflammatory response.

Improves Muscle Performance

If you didn't spend the last two decades or so in a cave, you might have heard that exercise is good for your health. When we train our muscles, the exercises actually cause a trauma to the skeletal muscle fibers. The trauma determines an intervention of the immune system that triggers an inflammatory response. The inflammation contains and repairs the damage, and helps clean up the waste products in the area.

And as you probably guessed by now, the autophagy mechanism helps clean up the waste products as well. This mechanism is actually the one responsible for a low to moderate immune response. If the autophagy wouldn't step in to clean up the waste products, the immune response would be greater and potentially dangerous.But the autophagy process improves our muscle performance in more ways than one.Even though they might not be useful, the damaged components of the cell still consume energy. By eliminating and recycling the damaged components, the autophagy helps the cell optimize its energy use and minimize its energy waste.

Can Help With Cancer Prevention

Chronic inflammation is one of the leading factors in cancer development. When a harmful particle abuses a cell, the body launches an inflammatory response. Sometimes, the inflammatory response cannot subdue the harmful agent in a timely manner. This leads to a chronic inflammation. Since the harmful agent is still present in the body, it can still produce toxins that can accumulate and lead to cancer.

Autophagy is helpful because it can help remove the harmful agent. Sometimes, even though it can't remove the agent, the cleanup process will prevent the toxin accumulation, lowering the stress the body faces. This allows it to suppress the cancer initiation.

Enhances Metabolic Efficiency

Autophagy eliminates all the cells' damaged components, preventing them from using energy needlessly. This will optimize the cells' energy use, which will make them stronger and more resilient. And a good thing about this cleanup process is that it's highly adaptable. If the body is facing a stressful situation, the autophagy mechanism will regulate the energy use by eliminating the cells' components that are unnecessary.

How to Induce Autophagy

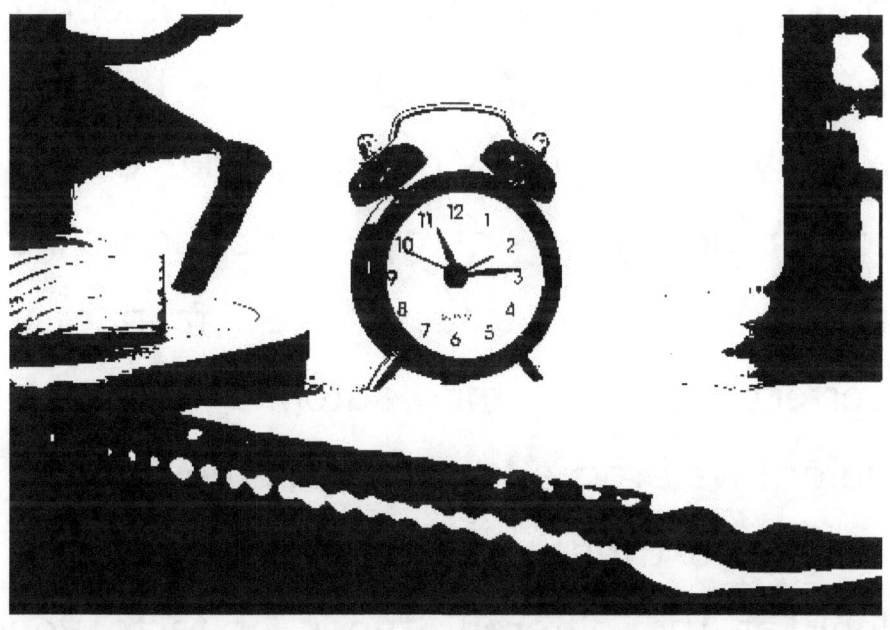

Now that we've listed the most important benefits of autophagy, let's take a look at how to stimulate this process.

Autophagy Fasting

Our bodies perceive fasting as stress. And that makes sense when you think about it. When you're fasting, you're hungry, moody, and your body will make efforts to optimize your energy distribution. And that's precisely what makes fasting a perfect trigger for autophagy. Now, before we proceed and explain how to use fasting to trigger autophagy, let's take a look at the different types of fasts you can choose from.

Long Fasts – These types of fasts require you to abstain from food for at least 24 hours.

Dry Fast – Despite its harshness, this is still a popular type of fast. The dry fast is extremely dangerous because you don't get to eat OR drink anything. Abstaining from drinking water is not advisable by any means. We do not recommend this fast. In fact, we recommend you avoid it, for your own sake.

Water Fast – Another popular type of fast, the water fast has been researched for its value in weight loss. This fast requires you to abstain from eating anything, but it allows and even recommends drinking water. Some people have adapted this fast, and they consume juices or protein shakes instead of water. While these methods might be effective for weight loss – even though multiple studies indicated that juicing is actually harmful to the body and is NOT indicated for weight loss – they are not true facts because you consume calories.

Long fasts promote weight loss and autophagy. A single 24-hour fast can reverse the loss of stem cell function, which will dramatically improve their regeneration capacities.

You might be wondering how long you have to fast to stimulate autophagy – well, most studies agree that a period of 24-hours would suffice. Some studies indicate that a fasting period of 16 hours would also stimulate the autophagy process, which suggests that time-restricted and intermittent fasting are viable options.

Even though some studies found that time-restricted and intermittent fasting are viable options to trigger autophagy, they are not as reliable as the long fasts. If you want to make sure you stimulate the process, abstain from eating for a period of 24 – 36 hours. Keep in mind that fasting is about avoiding calories. That doesn't mean you shouldn't drink water, tea, or coffee, as long as you don't add any sugar or other sweeteners to them.

Ketogenic Diet AUTOPHAGY

One of the benefits of the ketogenic diet is that it limits your calorie consumption without limiting your food intake. This diet requires you to consume at least 75 percent of your calories from fat and refrain from consuming more than ten percent from carbohydrates. Your body prefers to use the glucose extracted from carbohydrates as fuel, but if it doesn't find any carbs easily available, it changes its metabolic pathways and uses ketones extracted from fat as fuel instead.

Now, this shift might seem important to those who want to lose weight, but where does autophagy fit into this scenario?

Well, this shift actually happens naturally when we fast. The human body is highly adaptable. When we fast, our bodies look for other energy sources besides glucose, and they start breaking down fat to overcome starvation. This process is called ketogenesis. When the body is in a ketogenic state, the autophagy process is stimulated to optimize the cells' energy consumption and improve the body's energy output.

The ketogenic diet triggers the same process to help us lose weight. But the great thing about this diet is that you don't have to starve yourself to trigger ketogenesis. This makes the ketogenic diet a viable option for those who are unable to fast.

Exercise

Physical exercise stimulates the autophagy process. Exercise stimulated autophagy in multiple tissues and organs, such as the liver, pancreas, muscle, and adipose tissue. Surprisingly, exercise-induced autophagy in the cerebral cortex.

Even though this aspect is not fully understood at the moment, it strengthens researchers' belief that regular exercise could prevent the onset of neurodegenerative diseases such as Alzheimer's or Parkinson's. In addition, it seems like the exercise-induced autophagy helped with the development of new neurons and it helped improve the cognitive function. The process also optimized the energy consumption of the liver and pancreatic cells.

BENEFICIAL EFFECTS OF EXERCISE ON NAFLD

Changes in lifestyle such as weight loss and dietary modification have long been established as the first step in the management of NAFLD. Weight loss seems to independently improve hepatic function in NAFLD, although improved profile of intrahepatic lipids requires at least 3%–5% weight loss through physical activity and calorie control. Exercise alters various biochemical activities not only in the muscle, but also in the liver and adipose tissue. The muscle-liver cross talk in energy and metabolic balance also is inferred from the observation that the patients with CLD manifest a higher incidence of sarcopenia, a loss of muscle mass. A recent study further suggests a strong association between sarcopenia and NAFLD in both nonobese and obese subjects. The importance of muscle-liver cross talk also is implicated in a transgenic animal study where genetic ablation of myostatin, a TGF-β superfamily member that regulates skeletal muscle mass, ameliorated high fat diet–induced elevation of liver weight. Considering multiple benefits on the metabolic syndrome by increasing physical activity, it has been proposed that the skeletal muscle could be a pharmacological target for treating metabolic disorders including NAFLD.

How exercise directly or indirectly diminishes intrahepatic lipids independently of diet modification, however, remains unclear. The simplest view could be mobilization of hepatic lipids to the muscle to fuel muscular energy deficit during physical activity. Exercise increases glucose uptake in the muscles and concomitantly signals the liver to enhance glucose production to support continued energy expenditure.

The demand for increased gluconeogenesis further stimulates the degradation of intracellular lipids to provide mitochondrial substrates for β-oxidation. Besides enhancing free fatty acid oxidation in mitochondria, physical activity, particularly chronic aerobic exercise, also may reduce hepatic lipogenesis. In a high fat–fed mouse model, treadmill exercise substantially decreases the expression of sterol regulatory element-binding protein-1c, a transcription factor triggering triglyceride synthesis. Chronic consumption of high fat or high carbohydrate diet elevates levels of inflammatory cytokines such as tumor necrosis factor (TNF) α and interleukin-1β . We previously have shown that in the livers of old rats there was a significant increase in nuclear presence of nuclear factor κB and several other proteins, demonstrating an increased pro-inflammatory response. The age-associated increase in the upregulation of pro-inflammatory proteins was substantially attenuated in the livers of old animals exposed to long-term voluntary exercise by wheel running. Although physical exercise may attenuate hepatic inflammation by reducing pro-inflammatory cytokines, the mechanisms of anti-inflammatory benefits by exercise remain to be elucidated.

Using a mouse treadmill model, He et al.recently showed that physical activity stimulates autophagy in a wide range of tissues, including the skeletal muscle, heart, liver, pancreas, and adipose tissue. The exercise-mediated autophagy induction likely is to occur at the initiation step of autophagy through the dissociation of BECN1 from BCL2. Mice lacking three conserved phosphorylation sites of Thr69, Ser70, and Ser97 in the nonstructured loop of BCL2 failed to induce autophagy after exercise. Furthermore, these genetically modified animals were unable to run on a treadmill as long as their wild-type counterparts, implying that BECN1-dependent autophagy may be uniquely launched by exercise. Intriguingly, analysis of p62 and LC3-II/LC3-I, markers of autophagy induction, revealed that exercise also markedly increases autophagy in extramuscular tissues such as the liver and pancreas, although no apparent morphological or structural alterations were observed in hepatocytes and pancreatic β-cells from the mice expressing nonphosphoryltable BCL2. In particular, long-term exercise ameliorated high fat diet–induced glucose intolerance in wild-type mice but not in BCL2 mutant mice, substantiating the importance of autophagy in exercise-mediated cytoprotection against metabolic disorder.

Taken together, this study demonstrates that exercise is a natural stimulus of autophagy that can confer metabolic protection.How the muscle transduces an autophagy initiation signal to the liver is currently unknown. The skeletal muscle is an endocrine organ secreting a plethora of cytokines, chemokines, growth factors, hormones, and vasoactive factors, collectively termed myokines. Autophagy induction after physical training might involve these myokines. Myonectin or C1q/TNF-related protein 5 (CTRP5) is a nutrient-responsive myokine that enhances glucose uptake and stimulates fatty acid oxidation. This myokine often is released in response to feeding and insulin. Interestingly, exogenous administration of recombinant CTRP5 to the liver and cultured hepatocytes has been shown to prevent autophagy via activating mTOR pathway. Using a high fat diet rodent model, Lei et al. demonstrated that CTRP5-null animals exhibit reduced hepatic steatosis and improved insulin action, implying a negative correlation between CTRP5 and NAFLD onset. Intriguingly, aerorobic exercise has been reported to diminish levels of CTRP5 in humans. Although future studies are warranted to determine how this muscle-derived cytokine is delivered to and triggers autophagic signals in the liver, these studies suggest that hepatic autophagy could be modulated by the changes in CTRP5 levels after physical activity

Other myokines also might mediate autophagy stimulation in the liver. Irisin, an active form of the fibronectin type III domain containing 5 protein, is a newly identified exercise-induced myokine. Irisin activates AMPK signaling in hepatocytes and reduces intracellular triglyceride accumulation. Because AMPK is an essential player in autophagy initiation, irisin derived from the muscle might be an important signaling molecule that translocates to the liver and stimulates hepatic signaling of autophagy (Figure). However, it is important to note that despite numerous studies, large controversy still exists as to how much irisin increases after exercise in humans. Tandem mass spectrometric analysis of 10 individuals found that high intensity aerobic exercise increases the level of circulating irisin by 19%. Although statistically significant, this elevation is rather small. Future studies are required with larger populations of subjects to investigate how various exercise conditions affect irisin production in humans and how the liver interacts with this myokine released from the muscle.

Reduced calorie intake without malnutrition or calorie restriction (CR) has long been shown to effectively expand lifespan in various species including primates. One potential mechanism of CR-mediated benefit may be its induction of autophagy. Several studies have demonstrated that chronic or long-term CR facilitates protein turnover by activating multiple regulatory pathways of autophagy. For instance, CR acts on the upstream events of autophagy initiation by suppressing mTORC1 and stimulating AMPK, which in turn leads to ULK1 activation. Furthermore, CR enhances sirtuin 1 activity, an enzyme that induces autophagy through deacetylating multiple cellular targets. Although autophagy evidently is launched by either CR or exercise, ongoing controversies exist as to whether the combination of dietary intervention with exercise could provide greater benefits than CR or exercise alone

Although resistance exercise increases the strength and cross-sectional area of muscle fibers, endurance exercise, also known as aerobic exercise, augments the mitochondrial function and content of the muscle. Although either type of exercise profoundly influences cellular protein turnover, accumulating evidence indicates differential effects on protein homeostasis between resistance and endurance exercise. Within 24 h after acute endurance exercise, messenger RNA of key autophagy factors, including LC3, ATG4B, ATG12, BNIP3, and cathepsin L, is upregulated. A study with a mouse model of 40-min exercise duration showed that moderate-to-low intensity exercise rapidly promotes the phosphorylation of the residues of Ser317 and 555 of ULK1, while preventing mTORC1-dependent ULK1 phosphorylation, events indicative of autophagy initiation. It is, however, noteworthy that the increase in autophagy in response to a common endurance exercise is not always observed in other studies wherein animals are exposed to 50 to 90 min of tread mill exercise. This could imply that exercise duration may be an important factor contributing to autophagy induction in the muscle. Another important factor in endurance exercise–mediated autophagy induction is a feeding status before exercise. When autophagy onset during endurance exercise is compared between fast and fed state, stimulation of autophagy becomes more robust in the fasted state, as evidenced by a higher increase in LC3, BNIP3, and Parkin

In contrast with endurance exercise, a decrease in autophagy has been reported after resistance exercise. In humans, although resistance exercise reduces the lipidation of LC3-I, an integral event for autophagy induction, E3-ligase activity in the ubiquitin-proteasome pathway seems to be upregulated after this exercise regimen. Increased expression of class III PI3K has been reported after resistance exercise. However, because this kinase also is involved in multiple pathways other than autophagy, these studies do not necessarily reflect autophagy involvement in response to resistance exercise. Although current literatures favor nonessential roles of autophagy in strength and resistance exercise, future studies are needed to clarify better how autophagy is associated with this exercise regimen. It also is important to understand potential impacts of a combination of resistance and endurance exercise on muscle autophagy

EFFECTS OF MUSCLE AUTOPHAGY ON THE LIVER

Growing evidence supports the presence of a remote communication between individual organs. The skeletal muscles are a major provider of gluconeogenic and ketogenic amino acids during prolonged starvation in mammals. Because the liver is a primary tissue controlling both gluconeogenesis and ketogenesis and starvation is a powerful autophagy inducer in the liver and muscle as well, it is plausible to speculate that muscle autophagy could impact the liver directly or vice versa. Although defective autophagy in the muscle causes accumulation of intramyocellular triglycerides and enhanced autophagy facilitates removal of lipids from muscle cells, Takagi et al. recently demonstrated in tissue-specific ATG5 knockout mice that the mice lacking ATG5 in both the liver and muscle indeed exhibited the improvement of metabolic profile, compared with liver-specific knockout counterparts, suggesting that autophagy in the skeletal muscle metabolically may be distinct from that in the liver. In an independent study, skeletal muscle–specific ATG7 knockout mice also showed lower lipid accumulation and higher expression of β-oxidation–related genes, compared with control mice . Furthermore, when fed with high fat diet, these transgenic animals displayed lower expression of lipogenic genes in the liver and were protected from diet-induced obesity and insulin resistance. Because high fat diet markedly causes accumulation of lipid droplets in the autophagy-deficient livers, it is likely that metabolic outcomes after the onset of autophagy or lipophagy in the muscle may be different from those in the liver

Sleep

Even though most of us give up sleep to watch their favorite series, work more, or spend time with friends, our bodies function best when we respect their natural clocks or circadian rhythms. Our biological clock controls our sleep cycles, but it seems it controls the autophagy process as well.

Respecting our circadian rhythm is very important because it actually controls our metabolism. Our bodies order the production and release of hormones while we sleep. The lack of sleep is considered a stressful activity, and it has adverse effects on our health and wellbeing.

And sleep is also necessary to induce autophagy. The lack of sleep disturbs the autophagy process, and it slows it down considerably.

Autophagy boosting foods

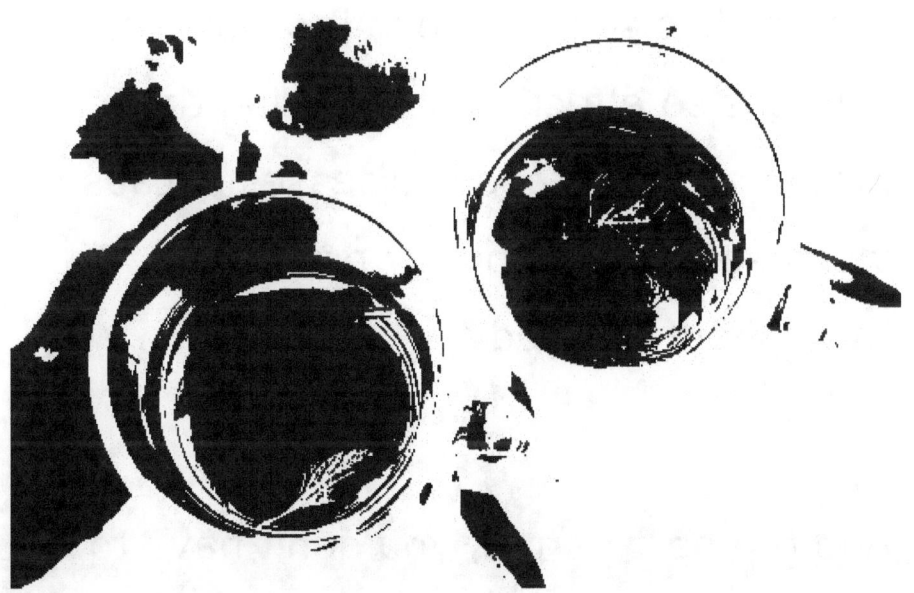

Eating certain foods can stimulate the autophagy process. Here is a list of the most efficient foods you can eat to induce this cleaning process.

Coffee

Several studies suggested that coffee consumption could inhibit several metabolic diseases. Now, it seems that coffee is so effective at reducing the incidence of metabolic diseases because it increases the autophagy process throughout the body.

And the best part is, you don't have to abuse caffeine to benefit from these effects. Scientists have noticed an increased autophagy in the heart, liver, and muscle cells after the consumption of a single coffee cup.

Ginger

Ginger consumption can induce autophagy. The active component of ginger, called 6-shogaol, can induce an autophagy process that's so powerful it can actually help destroy a type of lung cancer cells.

Green Tea

Some of the active ingredients found in green tea can stimulate the autophagy process in the liver cells. EGCG, a polyphenol commonly found in green and white tea can induce the autophagy in the liver. This process is helpful against inflammation, cancer, and liver damage.

Coconut Oil

Coconut oil contains a lot of ketones, the same components the body produces naturally when we're starving. By consuming these components through coconut oil, we trick the body into inducing autophagy without starving ourselves.

Reishi Mushroom

The Reishi mushroom has been used in Asian traditional medicine for centuries, which determined scientists to study its therapeutic effects. Recent studies suggest that the Reishi mushroom induces autophagy, which can produce anticancer effects in those who suffer from breast cancer.

*** Delicious recipe for **Autoph-Tea**, one of the easiest ways you can support the activation of autophagy in your cells

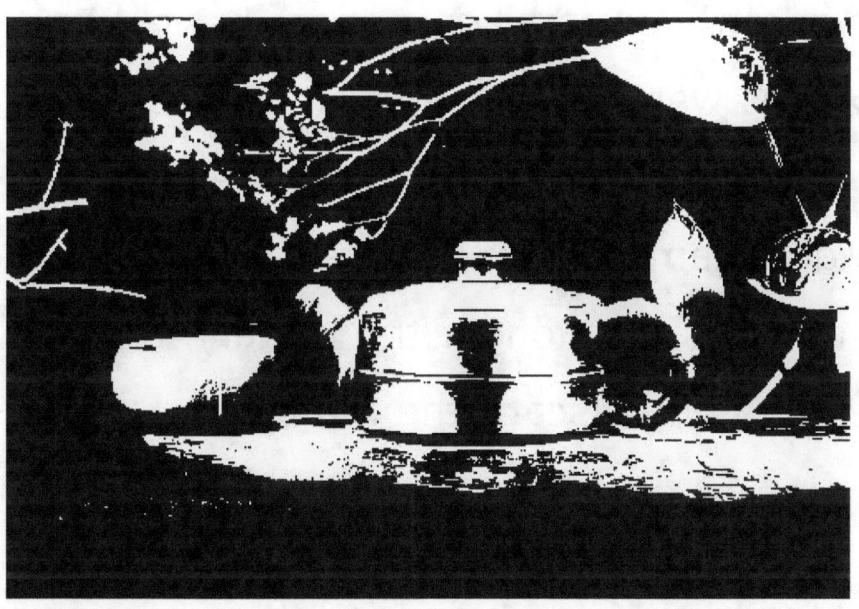

• 1 green tea bag

• 1 whole citrus bergamot Earl Grey tea bag

- 1 tablespoon raw coconut oil

- 1 cinnamon stick (Ceylon cinnamon)

- 1 teaspoon monk fruit powder (optional)

In a kettle or small saucepan, bring 1 to 1 ½ cups water to a boil. Pour the water into a large mug and add the tea bags and cinnamon stick. Let steep for at least 3 minutes (the longer the better), then remove and discard the tea bags.

Add the coconut oil and stir it in using the cinnamon stick.

Mix it all together for 20 to 30 seconds. You can also blend the tea to help mix the favors and emulsify the oil.

Take the overwhelm out of reclaiming your health...incorporate small ways like drinking Autoph-Tea daily to yield big results.

Natural Supplements That Boost Autophagy

The following natural supplements can also be used to induce autophagy

Resveratrol

Resveratrol is a compound commonly found in grapes, wine, and soy. This compound induces autophagy that can help inhibit breast cancer cells and can reduce the toxicity within the body.

Nicotinamide

Nicotinamide is a component of the vitamin B complex. Consuming this natural supplement can stimulate the autophagy process, which will reduce the pathologic accumulations that lead to the development of Alzheimer's disease.

Vitamin D

Vitamin D is synthesized naturally by our skin when it's exposed to sunlight. However, not many of us can expose our skin to the sun to produce vitamin D, especially in the cold season. This is why doctors recommend vitamin D supplementation.

Vitamin D can induce a powerful autophagy in the pancreatic cells, which can stimulate the insulin production and help prevent the onset of diabetes.

Melatonin

Melatonin is a hormone that plays an important role in the regulation of our circadian rhythm. Recent studies show that melatonin supplementation can induce autophagy in the brain, protecting it against cell injury. This could prevent several neuropsychiatric conditions.

Ginseng

Ginseng is one of the most popular natural supplements in the world. The ginseng root's active components induce autophagy and they have a protective role against breast cancer cells and melanoma.

The Genetics of Autophagy

Just like every other process in our body, autophagy is controlled directly and indirectly by genes. The genes that control this process determine how efficient it will be in collaborating with the immune system, and how well it will function as we grow older.

The Autophagy On/Off Switch

If autophagy is so efficient in protecting our bodies against harmful agents like bacteria, viruses, and cancer cells, why doesn't it make us immune to them?

Well, unfortunately, the natural autophagy process cannot keep up with the aging process. As our bodies grow older, our cells accumulate more and more debris inside them. The autophagy mechanism is triggered, and the lysosomes start cleaning up the cells. But they simply can't keep up with the workload.

Cells die continuously inside the body. The autophagy process cannot take place continuously in every part of the body. The active process always targets the cells that face the highest stress and works in a maintenance mode everywhere else.

For example, your skin cells face a high stress when you get a sunburn. Some of the cells die and trigger apoptosis, while others are damaged and trigger the autophagy. Sure, your damaged liver cells will still get fixed, but the body's focus is not on them at that moment. It needs to handle the skin burn first. That's the priority.

However, we can activate the autophagy mechanism at will. This can be accomplished in two ways. We can either consume foods or dietary supplements that induce the process, or we can produce some form of stress on the body and trigger it. Fasting and dieting are the easiest and healthiest ways to induce stress as a trigger for autophagy.

The Benefits Of Using Autophagy

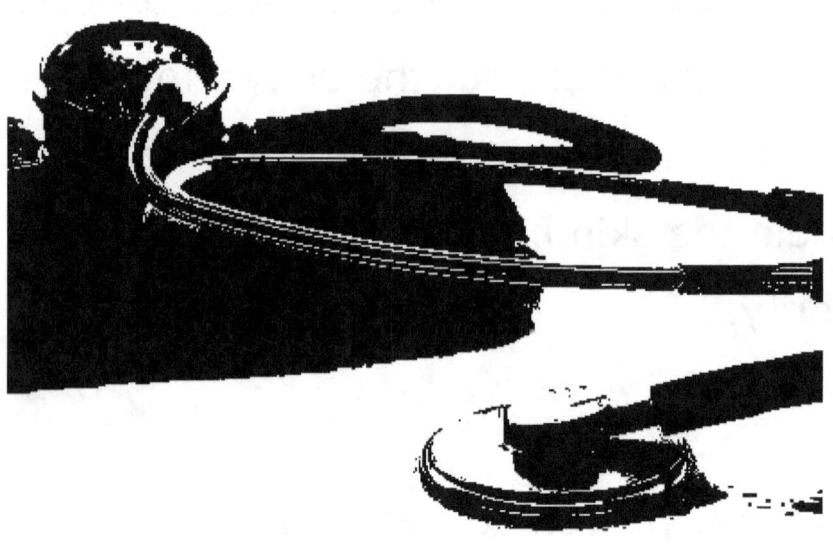

As you could see, inducing autophagy presents multiple possible benefits. While this topic is still under scientific scrutiny, most researchers agree that the autophagy process can help us lead better and healthier lives.

1. Autophagy may save your life.

Dramatic? Yes. But, scientifically accurate. Autophagy is an ancient mechanism whose main function is to preserve your life. During times of extreme stress, infection, or starvation, this process kicks in to maximize repair while minimizing damage. The combination of intermittent fasting (with some fat as fuel) while activating autophagy at the same time can both starve an infectious intruder of glucose, reduce inflammation so the immune system has an easier time taking action, and repair damage caused by both infection and inflammation. In short, animals evolved using autophagy to conserve energy and repair damage when energy became scarce, but it is also a critical part of the human immune system's ability to battle illness and reduce risk of cancer.

2. Autophagy may improve your quality and length of life.

Anti-aging benefits may sound too good to be true, but beauty really does run far deeper than the skin. Since the 1950s, scientists have known about the process of autophagy, but recent studies have revealed more about how it improves your cellular health. Instead of taking in new nutrients, cells undergoing autophagy recycle the damaged parts they have, remove toxic material and fix themselves up. When your cells repair themselves, they work better, and they can behave like younger cells. You may have heard or noticed that some people have a very different chronological (time) and biological (life) age. How much toxic damage a body has taken and how it has been able to repair plays a large role in these differences.

3. Autophagy helps your metabolism work better.

Autophagy is a process of taking out trash and replacing cell parts, like mitochondria. Mitochondria are your cellular engines. They burn fat and make ATP, your body's energetic currency. There is a lot of harsh toxic build up in mitochondria that can damage cells, and breaking them down proactively saves future wear and tear on your cells. Autophagy of other cell parts helps the entire cell work more efficiently not just to burn fuel but also to make proteins. Healthier cells work more efficiently.

4. Autophagy reduces risk of neurodegenerative diseases.

Many diseases of aging brains take so long to develop because they are the result of proteins in and around your brain cells that are misfolded and don't work right. Autophagy helps cells clean up the proteins that aren't doing their jobs and they are less likely to accumulate. For instance, in Alzheimer's disease autophagy removes amyloid, and in Parkinson's autophagy removes α-synuclein. There is a reason dementia is thought of hand-in-hand with diabetes: constant high blood sugar keeps autophagy from activating, making it difficult to keep these cells clear of clutter!

5. Autophagy helps regulate inflammation.

Autophagy promotes a "goldilocks" amount of inflammation by helping to boost or quell the immune response you need. Autophagy can increase inflammation when an invader is present by triggering your immune system to attack. Most of the time, autophagy decreases inflammation from your immune response by removing the signals (proteins called antigens) that are triggering it.

6. Autophagy helps us fight infectious disease.

As mentioned above, autophagy can help recruit an immune response when needed. Secondly, the process of autophagy can remove certain microbes directly from the inside of cells, such as Mycobacterium tuberculosis, or viruses, such as HIV. Autophagy can also remove the toxins created by infections, which is especially important for food-borne illness.

7. Autophagy improves muscle performance.

As you create microtears and inflame muscles during exercise, the muscles require repair. Energy demand increases.

Your muscle cells will respond to this by undergoing autophagy to reduce the energy required to use the muscle, degrade damaged components, and improve the balance of energy to reduce the risk of future damage.

8. Autophagy helps prevent cancer onset.

Autophagy can suppress processes that are pro-cancer like chronic inflammation, genome instability, and the DNA damage response. Mice that researchers have genetically engineered to have impaired autophagy have increased rates of cancer. As cancer progresses, it may activate autophagy to get alternative fuel or to hide from the immune system, though more research is needed. It is also unclear how much chemotherapy-induced damage to non-cancerous cells activates autophagy. In the future we may question how much damage chemotherapy does to cancer cells (killing them outright) versus to our own cells (activating autophagy to trigger an immune response that affects these cells). Again, more research is needed.

9. Autophagy improves your digestive health.

The cells that line your gastrointestinal tract are constantly asked to do work. In fact, a large part of your feces are your own cells! As a result of turning on autophagy, your digestive cells can repair and restore, clear themselves of junk, and reduce or activate the immune system as needed. Because a chronic immune response in the gut can overwhelm and inflame your bowels, a chance to rest, repair, and restore is critical to your gut health. Activate autophagy with a schedule that allows for an extended overnight fast and you can give your gut the space it needs to heal.

10. Autophagy improves your skin health.

The cells that you present to the world take a lot of damage from chemicals, air pollution, light, heat, cold, humidity changes, and physical damage. It's a wonder they don't look worse for wear! When your skin cells accumulate damage and toxins, they age in place. Even though you make new cells often, autophagy can help repair the existing ones so that you really glow! Skin cells, in particular, engulf bacteria that may damage the body, so it is very important to support them as they clear out the clutter. Learn more about at-home skin treatments and recipes to support your largest organ in my New York Times bestselling book Glow15 and on my website!

11. Autophagy may support a healthy weight.

Here are some benefits of autophagy that also support a healthy weight:

Autophagy requires fat-burning to be turned on but spares protein. On very long fasts, you will lose protein mass, but in shorter periods of fasting, you can activate autophagy, burn fat, spare protein, and get all the benefits of a leaner, fitter you.

Autophagy quells unnecessary inflammation. Chronic inflammation raises insulin, causing more weight storage– so less inflammation helps reduce insulin levels.

Autophagy reduces toxins in your cells. As long as you can excrete those toxins, they are less likely to need fat cells to store them.

Autophagy supports metabolic efficiency by repairing the parts of cells that make and package proteins and process energy, which is particularly helpful when cells need to switch to fat-burning for energy.

12. Autophagy (cell-eating) minimizes apoptosis (cell death).

Apoptosis is programmed cell death. Compared to autophagy, the death of a cell is messy and creates garbage to clean up. Your body triggers some inflammation to do the clean-up. The more cells that repair themselves before they become damaged beyond repair, the less effort your body puts into cleaning up old cells and making new ones. Less inflammation is involved in renewing tissues. You can use that energy to replace cells that need more constant renewal, like skin or digestive cells. While there are some cells that must be turned over a lot, not all cells require this. More repair with less cleanup is a great combination for success.

While autophagy has many health benefits, it is a repair response to stress and should not be on all the time. In my Glow15 Program, I share with you how to turn autophagy on and off inside your cells to get the best of both worlds!

AUTOPHAGY: THE NEW BIOLOGICAL STRATEGY FOR LONGEVITY

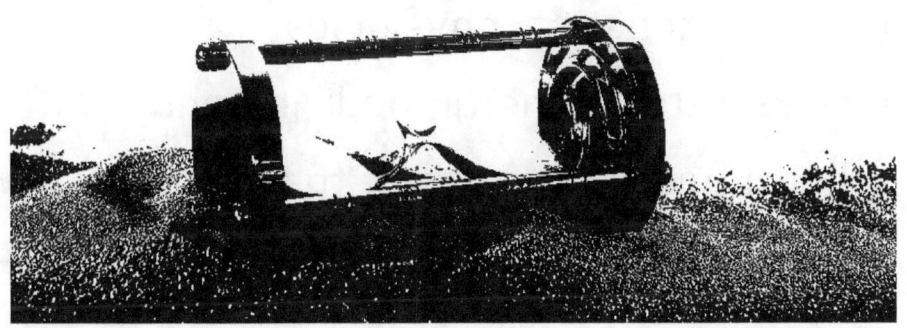

The research on the longevity of living beings is carried out in the field of biogerontology, that sector of biology that deals with knowing the natural mechanisms of aging, mechanisms that determine the life span of organisms (from invertebrates to humans) . Information on these processes (and on the possible possibility of modifying them to slow down the aging process and prolong the existence of individuals) involves a variety of biological disciplines (such as genetics, physiology, biochemistry, general medicine and others) and the results of the studies conducted (which have lasted more than a century generally on animal cells or whole organisms) seem to converge globally on two apparently antithetical general positions: the role of genetic predisposition to aging and the influence of the external environment on lifespan. While in the first case it would be the genes proper to an organism, with their functioning, the main ones responsible for its aging speed (and therefore its long or short duration of existence), in the second perspective to determine the individual differences of longevity would count of plus the lifestyle led by the body (food, disease, pollution, stress, etc.)

Since currently the majority of scholars tend to integrate the two cited proposals (rather than separate), many experts agree that to determine the actual life span of a living being contribute (to varying degrees) both its peculiar genetic component and his way of living (and therefore of eating, doing physical activity, and so on).

The study of the genetic components of longevity is enriched day by day with new information and discoveries (such as those concerning the telomerase enzyme), but it increasingly demonstrates the great complexity of the problem (the high number of genes "in play") , and, to the detriment of the easy hopes of increasing lifespan through pharmacologically targeted genetic manipulations, dangerous (and at the same time not easy to control) side effects emerge (at least for the moment). Therefore, until the roles of all the genes involved in the aging process are known in detail, the interventions aimed at modifying their functioning (for pro-longevity purposes) still appear premature and potentially dangerous.

On the other hand, on the other hand, over half a century of research has shown the prevalence of two fundamental factors capable of increasing life span: physical activity conducted by organisms and the reduction of calories consumed with the daily diet (calorie restriction). Most animal experiments on the effects of physical activity (moderate) agree on the beneficial effect, in terms of health and longevity, of physical exercise: the increase in this activity would result in a lower incidence of metabolic diseases , circulatory and other (in addition to greater longevity) in the subjects who practice it, compared to the more sedentary ones.

Similar results emerge from studies (mainly on rodents and primates) on calorie restriction: animals on a restricted diet of more than 30% of the calories normally taken at meals are significantly healthier and more long-lived than those who eat freely.

If for a long time scientists have not been able to clarify in detail the biological mechanisms underlying these two paradigms, recently in Italy (in Pisa) the research group of Professor Ettore Bergamini has contributed significantly to unraveling the mystery: the benefits for the health and longevity linked to the reduction of diet calories are intimately linked to a phenomenon inherent in all eukaryotic cells (including ours), that is cellular autophagy. This autophagy, and macroautophagy to be precise, is a phenomenon of recycling and repair of the damaged components of the cell (cytoplasmic proteins, membranes and organelles) due to the incessant harmful action carried out by free radicals (oxidative stress). These radicals, chemically unstable and highly reactive, are substances that are inevitably produced as a result of normal cellular metabolism, inflammation, stress, pollution, etc. and are capable of attacking and seriously damaging the structures of the cell, if not effectively counteracted. itself (like macromolecules and organelles). The latter can avoid succumbing by accelerating its rhythm of division (reproduction), but will thus more quickly reach the condition of senescence (the number of possible divisions is limited) and therefore to premature death. Macroautophagy is thus a rescue system: the oxidized cytoplasmic proteins, the old and damaged organelles (such as the mitochondria, the "energy centers" of the cells) and other important structures are thus isolated from the rest of the cellular cytoplasm and incorporated into said membranous vesicles autophagosomes. Subsequently these autophagosomes fuse into the cytoplasm with lysosomes (organelles full of "digestive" hydrolytic enzymes) which thus pour their content into the autophagosomes themselves and allow the enzymatic demolition (digestion) of the material previously sequestered there. In this way, the cells can, for example, degrade damaged proteins (autophagic proteolysis) by then recycling many "building materials" (amino acids) for energy or reconstruction purposes. These cells, therefore, having repaired the damage and being renewed in their fundamental structures, can slow down the rhythm of division and therefore live longer. Macroautophagy is normally mildly induced during the first 24 hours of fasting (a form of short-term caloric restriction) of animals (laboratory rats) mainly in the internal organs (such as the liver), but is totally suppressed in the period immediately following at meals. The Bergamini team has discovered that autophagy tends, however, to naturally weaken as animals age (perhaps due to the progressive inevitable accumulation of oxidative stress damage), but it can be significantly intensified even in older animals through the use (coupled with fasting) of particular drugs called anti-hypolithic drugs, capable of blocking the release of fat in the blood (for energy purposes) from adipose tissue. Pharmacologically treated rodents in this way were much less subject to age-related diseases (cardio-vascular problems, diabetes, tumors) than untreated animals of the same age that continued to feed at will (the controls). The first experiments with the method also started on human volunteers and, according to Bergamini himself, show very encouraging results.

hormone insulin (a pathological characteristic present in many elderly people), a precursor to diabetes and, in general, to cellular aging.

In essence, science is now able to fully re-evaluate ancient health precepts (a brief, occasional fast and frequent and moderate physical activity) to be performed at any age and to be used, for preventive purposes, from an early age, to try to stay in health and to slow aging, at least in part.

Cell death: difference between necrosis, apoptosis and autophagy

Cell death can be implemented in various ways and for different causes (physiological or pathological).

Apoptosis

Apoptosis is a type of programmed cell death that occurs physiologically and / or pathologically in response to different stimuli: physiological stimuli for apoptosis can occur in:

selection of cells in tissues in active proliferation (for example, selection of lymphocytes that respond to self in the bone marrow)

cell selection during embryogenesis

elimination of cells that are no longer useful (such as lymphocytes after the removal of an antigen).

Pathological stimuli that induce apoptosis are generally due to: DNA damage (unrepairable), abnormal folding of proteins, infections. The activation of apoptosis can occur through two pathways that converge on the same effector proteins (caspases). The most common way is called intrinsic or mitochondrial because it is mediated by these organelles: the control of apoptosis is guaranteed by the balance of the anti- and pro-apoptotic signals by proteins called BCL. These form channels on the mitochondrial surface that regulate their permeability: the main antiapoptotic factor is BCL2, while the most important proapoptotic BCLs are BAX and BAK. In reality these molecules act by dimerization and the prevalence of dimers leads to the apoptotic cell. If the action of BCL2 prevails over the others, the cell does not undergo apoptosis but if proteins called BH3only sensors of cellular stress intervene, the BAX and BAK channels open and let out the mitochondria proapoptotic enzymes that activate the caspases (for example the cytochrome c). the caspase activated in the intrinsic pathway is caspase 9 while caspases 8 and 10 are involved in the extrinsic pathway (of which the effector caspase is 3); the latter begins with binding to specific receptors on the cell membrane of death signals including TNFa, TNFb, FADD and FAS. The link between FAS and its ligand (FASL / CD95) is a coreceptor in the link between cytotoxic T lymphocytes and the corresponding APC. The interaction between these death signals and their receptors activate the intracellular procaspases 8 and 10 and the effector phase begins.

This involves the activation by the caspases of endonucleases that break the DNA and the degradation of the cytoskeleton by the caspases themselves. The residues of the dead cell form the so-called apoptotic bodies that are phagocytosed because they express molecules (usually intracellular) on the membrane that are recognized by macrophages.

Necrosis

Necrosis occurs only in pathological conditions when cellular damage is not reversible. Under conditions of hypoxia or even of ischemia (which causes more serious damage because the cell is also deficient in nutrients due to anerobic metabolism), the reduction of oxidative phosphorylation leads to a depletion of ATP and a consequent malfunction of the sodium-potassium-ATP dependent pump. Since the transit of ions into and out of the cell is compromised, the cell itself and the organelles increase their size due to osmotic swelling; not only: the incoming $Ca2+$ is increased and this determines the activation of different enzymes that degrade both the DNA and the cellular membrane which at this point disintegrates forming myelinated figures typical of necrosis and causing cell rupture. The release of intracellular enzymes can lead to damage to the surrounding tissue.

Various types of necrosis can be distinguished based on the morphology of the damaged tissue: coagulative necrosis, colliquative, fibrinoid, caseosa, gangrenous, steatonecrosis.

Coagulative necrosis is a type of necrosis generally resulting from ischemic damage due to obstruction of a vessel; in this type of necrosis the architecture of the tissue is generally preserved (in the first days, after which the cellular debris is phagocytized) because there is the denaturation of proteolytic enzymes which therefore cannot fulfill their function of degradation of structural proteins. An area of coagulative necrosis (following ischemia) is called infarction.

Colliquative necrosis is typical of the outbreak of bacterial infection and ischemia of the brain. Necrotic tissue is liquid and viscous because cellular debris is digested. The presence of dead leukocytes in the necrotic tissue gives it a yellowish color, in this case the liquid is called pus.

Gangrenous necrosis refers mainly to the limbs that present a blood supply deficit (and therefore a picture of coagulative necrosis). If the gangrene of the limbs overlaps a bacterial infection, the necrosis assumes the characteristics of a colliquative form for which one speaks of wet gangrene.

Caseous necrosis owes its name to the whitish appearance and the fragile consistency of the necrotic tissue; it is typical of the tuberculosis infection in which there is the formation (above all at the pulmonary level) of a complex with a central necrotic area surrounded by giant Langhans cells (macrophages morphologically transformed into epithelioid cells merge to form giant cells) and lymphocytes, called granuloma.

Steatonecrosis indicates areas of adipocyte necrosis often due to secretion of pancreatic lipases in the organ or peritoneal cavity (acute pancreatitis). The fat cells break and the triglycerides that release the fatty acids escape, which react with calcium forming whitish deposits visible in the organ concerned with a process called fat saponification.

Fibrinoid necrosis is typical of type III hypersensitivity reactions (mediated by immune complexes) in which the deposition and accumulation of antigen-antibody complexes and fibrous tissue inflames and damages the vessel walls, forming a pink-colored thickening around the clearly visible vessel under the microscope.

Autophagy

Autophagy is a process that the cell generally puts into practice in the event of nutrient deficiency; provides phagocytosis of its own organelles that are included in autophagic vacuoles that merge with lysosomes. Defective organelles and proteins are sequestered in double-membrane vesicles, autophagosomes:

induction: it is regulated by mTOR, a kinase that acts as a sensor of available energy levels and amino acids.

autophagosome formation: cytoplasmic material of various nature is incorporated into the autophagosome thanks to enzymes

recognition and fusion of the lysosome autophagosome: ensured, by different proteins including SNARE (membrane proteins that favor the attachment of vesicles);

demolition of the autophagic body: the content of the autophagolisosome is degraded by lysosomal hydrolases.

www.ingramcontent.com/pod-product-compliance
Lightning Source LLC
Chambersburg PA
CBHW072205280526

45788CB00002B/885